GERD Diet And Cookbook

"the new complete guide to prevent, treat and cure GERD, reflux acid, gastric acid with natural remedies. Meal plan with over 60 delicious quick and easy recipes"

Charles Thompson

The trademarks that are used are without any consent, and the publication of the trademark is without permission or backing by the trademark owner. All trademarks and brands within this book are for clarifying purposes only and are the owned by the owners themselves, not affiliated with this document.

Contents

Introduction 7

Chapter 1: Gastro-Esophageal Reflux Disease 8

    Causes 8

    Symptoms 10

    Treatments.. 11

    Risks and complications 13

Chapter 2: Prevention from GERD 14

    Foods to eat and avoid.. 14

    Impact of Exercise.. 15

    Lifestyle changes.. 16

Chapter 3: Recipes for breakfast 18

Chapter 4: Recipes for starter 28

Chapter 5: First dishes 38

Chapter 6: Main courses 49

Chapter 7: Recipes for Side dish 58

Chapter 8: Recipes for dessert... 68

Chapter 9: Drinks&Shakes... 79

Conclusion.. 87

Introduction

GERD also called gastric reflux or stomach acid and is a digestive system disorder. It can damage the esophagus, and heartburn is the main symptom of this condition. The esophagus is used for swallowing, and the disease occurs when the acid contained in the stomach returns through the esophagus and inflames it. If you have acid reflux, you may develop a sour or bitter taste in the mouth, and it may cause you to regurgitate food or liquid from the stomach.

One of the causes of GERD is poor nutrition, little variety of diet, little physical activity, lack of sleep, and stress. The best way to treat GERD symptoms is a radical change in lifestyle without smoking and alcohol. Follow a diet and exercise; they can help overcome acid reflux and improve their digestive health.

Studies have shown that between 21 and 40% of people suffer from heartburn. More than 60 million adult Americans suffer from heartburn at least once a month. Although acid reflux occurs in both women and men, men have been shown to have more GERD symptoms.

This book will provide you with many helpful tips on GERD, causes, symptoms, and numerous recipes for getting back to eating without pleasure. That annoying post-meal heartburn. In addition to a healthy diet, we will give particular attention to the correct lifestyle made of sports activities, the importance of sleeping, and reducing stress.

Chapter 1: Gastro-Esophageal Reflux Disease

Gastroesophageal reflux disease is often caused by reflux into the esophagus of stomach contents and intestinal gases that generate gastroesophageal reflux. This leads to heartburn or throat burning. Occasional small refluxes are considered physiological, for example, once a week, but if the symptom is repeated several times during the week, medical assistance must be requested.

Causes

GERD is caused due to multiple factors. GERD is caused by numerous factors. It is important to know and identify these reasons and problems. When you are aware of the causes, it is easier to change your lifestyle and improve yourself.
Here are the main causes of GERD:

Obesity

Obesity is a clinical condition in which the subject has significant accumulations of body fat. This can compromise vital functions and lead to a deterioration in the quality of life. Weight gain can cause problems with bones, body resistance, heart performance, blood circulation, and organ activities. The obese person has an increased abdominal circumference and therefore, an elevated abdominal pressure, which favors the ascent of gastric juices into the esophagus and promotes sphincter incontinence.

Alcohol

Alcohol is another important cause of GERD. Alcohol is, in fact, already dangerous in itself on people's health. It has been observed that high consumption of alcoholic beverages not only causes acid reflux but increases the risk of a pre-cancerous lesion of the esophagus and the tumor itself.

Smoke

Smoking is one of the biggest causes of GERD. Smoking affects not only the lungs but also the stomach because nicotine stimulates acid secretion. The combined effect of caffeine and nicotine causes an even higher increase in gastric acidity.

Low physical activity

As mentioned before, overweight and the consequent increase in the abdominal part is a cause of GERD, so a little physical activity during the week is good for you. You train correctly, with a specific program to your fitness, also following a specific nutritional plan. A healthy diet associated with exercise will be your allies in alleviating symptoms and reducing the probability of complications; your overall health will improve, and your quality of life will definitely have a positive turnaround.

Diet does not vary

Poor variety in the diet can have a negative effect on your overall health, and GERD can be caused by poor food options. If you consume junk food, snacks, soft drinks, high-fat foods, you may experience acid reflux.

Bad habits and incorrect posture

GERD can also occur from bad habits such as incorrect posture while eating, such as eating while lying down. Another bad habit is to go to lie on a bed or on the sofa after each meal. It is advisable to take a short walk after eating or at least not to go to bed immediately.

Pregnancy

GERD is one of the most common ailments in pregnancy because of hormonal changes and the position of the fetus. Usually, this is a problem that mostly affects the past three months.

Medications

Medications can lead to GERD as a side effect, including nonsteroidal anti-inflammatory drugs, aspirin, and some antibiotics.

Symptoms

Being aware of the symptoms is essential for healthy living, and starting to understand that we are suffering from GERD. As soon as we feel the symptoms of acid reflux, we must immediately act accordingly to avoid even serious complications. Here are a few major symptoms of gastric acid reflux to consider:

-Heartburn is the most common symptom. It appears as a burning sensation under the chest bone. Pain is caused by irritation of the lining of the esophagus due to the passage of acid that has risen from the stomach.

-Bitter in the back of the mouth and throat

-Burning throat in the upper part

-Even bloody and painful nausea and vomiting in severe cases

-GERD can cause very dark and bleeding stools, accompanied by burning

-Prolonged hiccups accompanied by burning and pain in the throat.

-Feeling that food is stuck in the throat.

-Difficulty in swallowing food, with pain and burning

-Sore throat, a dry cough can occur in the early stages.

-Halitosis and dental erosion are other main symptoms of GERD.

GERD can begin to present itself from the simple burp to the bloody vomit; therefore, one should not take to read these symptoms listed above, even the banalest. It is essential to identify these symptoms initially and to take immediate measures to quickly resolve these problems. Each of the above symptoms does not necessarily address all of them at once, but the symptoms are likely to occur from time to time. So it is important to pay attention to the initial symptoms as well. Sometimes you may have these problems along with other medical conditions, so be sure to discuss them with your doctor first.

Treatments

GERD is one of the most common digestive disorders involving millions of people around the world. When gastric reflux is not treated properly, it can produce hiatal hernia. It prevents the functioning of the diaphragm regulating valve, which has the task of controlling the flow of food and keeping food in the stomach. You should not underestimate the symptoms in order not to have complications later in your life. It is necessary to chase after treatments. As soon as possible.
Here is some treatment option:

Lifestyle

Sometimes simply changing your lifestyle is enough to get better in many health conditions. Specifically for GERD, you have to avoid some habits that many people in the world have, including:
stop smoking
abuse of alcohol
Eat quickly by chewing a little
follow a light diet with few or no spices
eat small meals and at intervals of time
lose weight
avoid chewing gum
bedtime
Dress in tight clothes
Perform substantial physical efforts immediately after meals
avoid bedtime immediately after eating

Natural treatments

There are some natural remedies for Gerd that include easily available supplements and herbs. However, they may be useful in combination with what your doctor recommends for GERD
Below is a list of herbs and supplements:

- Ginger root

  is one of the most common natural supplements for stomach problems. It relaxes the muscles in the esophagus and calms the digestive tract. Ginger also improves digestion and consequently helps reduce GERD or reflux because food and acid do not persist in the stomach.

- Licorice root
calms the stomach. It reduces inflammation of the lining of the esophagus and stomach, which is caused by GERD. It stimulates the body's natural defense mechanisms and is a natural anti-inflammatory.

- Lavender
its antispasmodic properties it is known to promote proper digestion and to limit the presence of gas in the gastrointestinal level. It is mainly used as an infusion.

- Chicory
the root can be a very useful digestive aid for people who have GERD. Chicory is also effective for relieving reflux pain because it helps relax the stomach.

- Antioxidants
antioxidant vitamins A, C, and E are recognized for their potential in preventing GERD. Vitamin supplements are usually used if not enough nutrients are received from food. A blood test can help determine which nutrients your body needs. Your doctor may also prescribe a multivitamin.

- Melatonin
as the "sleep hormone," melatonin is a hormone produced in the pineal gland. This gland is located in the brain. Melatonin is primarily known for helping initiate sleep.

- Aloe vera
in reducing the main reflux symptoms

Medications

- In the early stages of GERD, there are some medications you can use, so remember that you need to consult your doctor before undertaking any drug treatments. With medications, the

  aim is to reduce esophageal acidity, neutralizing the acid produced, or inhibiting its upstream production. There are different types of medications for gastroesophageal reflux (antacids, histaminergic receptor blockers, proton pump inhibitors) If not in serious cases, it is always to avoid taking them before using them and triggering the vicious circle. It would be good to consider other ways: diet, lifestyle, exercise, reduction of stress, and cigarette smoking. Make sure to consult the physician in severe cases for the medication prescription and regular checkups.

Risks and complications

If you underestimate the problem and delay with treatments, you can chase complications and risks.

Potential complications of GERD include:

- Esophageal stenosis, which occurs when the esophagus narrows or narrows
- Esophagitis (inflammation of the esophagus)
- Esophageal cancer, which affects a small portion of people with Barrett's esophagus
- Barrett's esophagus, which involves permanent changes to the lining of your esophagus
- Erosion of tooth enamel, gum disease.
- Asthma, chronic cough or other breathing problems

It is essential to solving the problem in the first phase to have adequate and easy-to-perform treatment, thus avoiding reaching more extreme solutions.

Chapter 2: Prevention from GERD

Yes, prevention is better than cure. You need to make sure you take some essential precautions that will help you live a healthy life. GERD is not caused by external factors such as viruses or infections but only by a wrong daily routine. With a little attention, it is quite easy to follow the prevention guide for GERD related problems.

Foods to eat and avoid

Most of the problems caused by GERD are related to poor nutrition, so it is necessary to follow a healthy and light diet. Eating correctly is the best method to prevent gastric reflux and allow you to have positive and tangible results in a short period. Now let's see how healthy food can become a valuable ally for prevention, and we will find out what foods to eat and avoid.

What not to eat

Avoid high-fat foods. These are difficult to digest, and this means they stay in the stomach longer. When foods slow down digestion, the chances of them returning to the esophagus increase, leading to reflux. To avoid this situation, you need to avoid foods such as:

- Animal fat such as lard, bacon, hamburger, pork fat cuts, cold cuts, hot dog, etc
- High-fat snacks that do not have much nutritional value, such as chips, candy, or ice cream.
- Fried foods such as chips, vegetable fries and fried chicken
- salmon, octopus, cuttlefish, mussels, clams, etc.

Protein foods raw or overcooked come:

- Ragout or similar
- Carpaccio, tartare, sushi, etc.
- Braised

Eat less acidic foods:

- Tomato and juice
- Citrus fruits and juice.
- Vinegar

High-calorie foods that can promote overweight:

- Very seasoned foods
- Cheeses
- pasta in an abundant portion

Spices and flavorings
- Chili pepper
- Onion and garlic(In ample quantities)
- Pepper
- All carbonated drinks.

The techniques not recommended are:
- Brazing
- Frying in a pan
- Stewing

Foods to eat

The following are the foods that must be part of the diet daily to prevent GERD:
- Among the recommended meats there are: chicken, rabbit, turkey, defatted pork or beef muscle, etc
- Among the fishery products: cod, anchovies, sea bream, sea bass, tuna fillet, prawns, etc.
- Among the cheeses: lean ricotta, light spreadable cheese, cottage cheese.
- Among legumes, cereals and derivatives, choose those with medium or low fiber content.
- fruits and vegetables

The recommended cooking techniques are:
- Steam-powered
- In a pressure cooker
- Boil in water
- Baked
- Grilled
- In a pan over low heat.

By following these dietary guidelines, you will take a big step forward to prevent GERD and have a healthy life.

Impact of Exercise

In the prevention of GERD, physical activity has a significant impact; as it is done after 2/3 hours after the main meal, it will consume all or part of the energy consumed by the food. It will also help you have faster digestion and consequently avoid acid reflux.

Weight reduction

Overweight or obesity are some of the reasons that can lead to GERD. Regular physical activity will lead to a decrease in weight associated with the correct diet. In general, reducing weight will help you have a better quality of life.

An active mind and healthy body

An excellent physical activity routine is an excellent combination of body and mind. With daily training, you will consume a lot of your strength and release a lot of the tension you have. With the effort due to a workout, our brain will release the stress hormone, and this will make for a good night's sleep.

Activate the repair muscles

Exercise and exertion activate the repairing muscles in the body, which help reduce internal and external inflammation. Exercise helps manage this painful condition and enables the body to repair damaged cells.

Lifestyle changes

To prevent GERD, it is necessary to make changes to your lifestyle, as mentioned in the previous pages. These changes not only help prevent the acid reflux problem but will also give you a better life and avoid further health problems.

Eat healthily

Healthy eating is the top priority. If you eat fatty foods, refined sugars must be replaced immediately. These foods must be consumed very rarely, only in rare situations. It is necessary to introduce healthy and light food among your food options to avoid such problems.

Plan your meals

Organizing your meals is essential for the prevention of GERD. Waiting too much between meals is never healthy because it leads to massive

meals and consequently, prolonged digestion. It is advisable to make small meals, eat little, and often with meals scheduled with specific intervals that reduce the risk of GERD.

Do not sleep immediately after a meal

Going to sleep shortly after eating is a bad habit that must be eliminated. The possibility of acid reflux increases as the position taken when sleeping does not guarantee proper digestion.

Maintain a balance between food options

Changing lifestyles does not mean abandoning all food options. Some foods should be favored over others, but the important thing is knowing how to balance food options and not just eating the same things all the time. Make sure you have many choices in your diet. That will help you have the right food balance.

Sleep well

Sleep is essential for digestion and stomach food to function well. Sleep is vital to allow digested food and stomach to work well. Make sure you sleep well at least between 7/8 hours. Sleeping little will make you feel tired and will not encourage you to want to exercise.

Do not stress yourself

Stress and anxiety can affect the proper functioning of the digestive system. Anxiety and stress have effects that fall on the stomach. A stressed brain negatively affects the general function of the organism.

Chapter 3: Recipes for breakfast

1) Maple syrup pancakes

Ingredients:
- **Butter vegetable 25 g**
- **00 flour 125 g**
- **Medium eggs 2**
- **Fresh whole milk 200 g**
- **Baking powder for cakes 6 g**
- **Brown sugar 15 g**
TO SEAL:
Maple syrup to taste

We begin the preparation of pancakes by melting the butter on shallow heat, then let it cool. Meanwhile, divide the egg whites from the yolks. Pour the yolks into a bowl and beat them with a hand whisk, then add the melted butter at room temperature and the milk flush, continuing to mix with the whisk. Whisk the mixture until it becomes clear. Add the yeast to the flour and sift everything in the bowl with the egg mixture, mix with the whisk to blend. Now whip the egg whites that you have kept aside, pouring the sugar little by little, and when they are white and frothy, gently add them to the egg mixture, with movements from top to bottom, to avoid disassembling them. Heat over medium heat (not high; otherwise you will not give the dough time to rise well during cooking, and the pancakes will become too dark) a large non-stick pan (preferably with a thick bottom) and, if necessary, grease with a little butter to spread on the surface with the help of kitchen paper. Pour a ladle of preparation into the center of the saucepan; there will be no need to spread it. When bubbles begin to appear on the surface, and the base will be golden, turn it on the other side using a spatula, as if it were a crepe or an omelet, then brown the other side in turn, after which the pancake will be ready. Continue with the rest of the dough, and gradually arrange the pancakes on a serving plate, stack them one on top of the other. About 12 pancakes should form with these doses. Serve them hot and sprinkled with maple syrup. You can accompany the pancakes with fresh fruit or sugar of your taste.

2) Muffin with chocolate drops
Ingredients:
- **Vegetable butter at room temperature 125 g**
- **almond flour 265 g**
- **135 g brown sugar**
- **Skimmed milk at room temperature 135 g**
- **Eggs (about 2) at room temperature 110 g**
- **Dark chocolate drops 100 g**
- **Vanilla bean 1**
- **1 tsp frosted bicarbonate**
- **Add a pinch of salt**
- **Baking powder 1**

To prepare the muffins with chocolate chips worked with the electric whisk butter, left to soften at room temperature for at least an hour previously, with the sugar, until obtaining a frothy and creamy mixture. Then cut a vanilla bean and scrape the seeds using the back of a knife. Pour the latter into the bowl with butter and sugar. Operate the whips again and add the eggs, also at room temperature, one at a time in this way the ingredients will not untie. Now sift the flour, baking powder, and baking soda directly into the bowl with the mixture. Also, add a pinch of salt and operate the whisk again to incorporate the powders. You will notice that the dough will become more consistent, then dilute it with milk at room temperature poured flush. At this point, the mixture will be soft and compact. Add 80 grams of chocolate chips and mix them with a spatula to incorporate them. Then transfer the mixture into a disposable bag without nozzle; in this way, you can do a cleaner job; otherwise, use a spoon as well. Place the paper cups in a muffin pan and fill them 2/3 full, leaving less than an inch from the surface.

Each muffin will have to weigh approximately 70 grams. Pour the remaining 20 drops of chocolate over the cupcakes and bake in a preheated oven at 180 ° for 18-20 minutes in static mode (otherwise at 160 ° for 13-15 minutes if the oven is ventilated). At this point, your chocolate chip muffins are ready to be enjoyed.

3) Yoghurt plum cake

Ingredients:
- **00 flour 300 g**
- **Eggs (about 5) 300 g**
- **Light butter 200 g**
- **200 g powdered sugar**
- **Low-fat yogurt 150 g**
- **Potato starch 50 g**
- **Powdered yeast for cakes 15 g**
- **Vanilla bean seeds 1**
- **Salt up to 4 g**

FOR MOLDS
- **Butter to taste**
- **00 flour to taste**

To prepare the yogurt plumcake, equip yourself with a mixer equipped with fairly powerful and capacious blades. Place the cubed butter, the seeds of the vanilla bean, the eggs and the flour in the container yogurt, icing sugar, salt, yeast, and starch. Work at maximum speed for about 4 minutes. In the meantime, grease and flour two 16x8 cm slightly flared molds. As soon as you have obtained a homogeneous mixture, transfer it into the molds. Now dip a blade of a knife, first in the melted butter and then in the center of the two plumcakes. This will ensure uniform growth in cooking. Now put the plumcake in a preheated static oven, and they will have to cook in 2 phases: first at 185 ° for 15 minutes, then at 165 ° for 30 minutes.

As soon as they are cooked, take them out of the oven and let them cool completely. At this point, turn them out and decorate them with icing sugar, and your yogurt plumcakes are ready to taste.

4) Vegetable tart

Ingredients:

- 1 pack of puff pastry of about 300 g
- 2 zucchini
- 4 potatoes
- 4 eggs
- 30 g of grated cheese
- basil
- chives
- extra virgin olive oil
- salt

To make the vegetable tart, start cutting the zucchini. Cut the two ends of the zucchini and cut into slices of about 5mm thick. Salt them slightly and let them drain in a colander. Peel the potatoes, wash and dry them, then cut as if you should make some fried chips by transferring them to a pan in which you have heated two tablespoons of oil.

Brown the potatoes and cook them for 10 minutes. Remove from the heat and put them on paper towels. In the same pan, place the well-dried zucchini and prepare it by turning it often for 15 minutes. In the meantime, beat the eggs. Cook the zucchini, put them in a bowl, add the potatoes and mix everything with the beaten eggs, the grated cheese, the basil, chopped and salted chives.

Brush a tart pan with oil and lay the puff pastry on it. Distribute the filling prepared evenly and bake in a hot oven at 200 ° for about 25 minutes. Then leave the vegetable tart to rest for about ten minutes and serve.

5) Potato omelette

Ingredients:

- **Eggs 6**
- **Potatoes 500 g**
- **Parmesan cheese 100 g**
- **Parsley to taste**
- **Salt to taste**
- **Seed oil to taste**

To make the potato omelet, first, put some water in a pan and bring to the boil. In the meantime, peel the potatoes and slice them. Now boil the potatoes for about 5 minutes. When cooking the potatoes finely chopped parsley. Now pour the eggs into a bowl, the chopped parsley, the grated cheese, and then salt At this point, mix to mix the ingredients. Drain the potatoes that have finished cooking, let them cool, and then add them to the egg mixture. Now go to cooking: in a pan heat a drizzle of seed oil, and once it is hot, pour the mixture. Cover with the lid and cook over moderate heat for 15 minutes, turning the pan occasionally. When the surface is not very soft but still damp, turn the omelet over the lid, rotating the pan upside down with a decisive and rapid movement. Slide the omelet back into the pan to cook the other side, cover again with the lid and continue cooking for another 5 minutes. After this time, the omelet will be ready. You can serve it hot or cold.

6) Apple heart biscuits

Ingredients:
- an egg
- 100 g of cane sugar
- half a bag of yeast
- wholemeal flour to taste
- a coffee glass of extra virgin olive oil
- grated orange peel

For the apple filling
- 3 apples
- 2 teaspoons of powdered ginger
- the juice of half a lemon
- 2 tablespoons of brown sugar

In a bowl, put the egg, brown sugar, grated orange peel, and olive oil. Mix the ingredients with a fork in a circular and continuous pattern until you get a homogeneous and creamy mixture. Stir in the yeast and mix. At this point, add the sifted flour a little at a time, always mixing it with a fork in the bowl. You will see the dough gradually transform, acquire body and shape while remaining soft. For the recipe's success, this is an important step: consider mixing the flour at the rate of a spoon at a time until your liquid and creamy dough become more compact but not hard. Transfer it to a lightly floured pastry board and knead. When it no longer sticks to your hands, your pastry will be ready. Give it a ball shape and place it in the refrigerator for 30 minutes.

7) Apple muffin

Ingredients:

- **Apples 310 g**
- **00 flour 300 g**
- **Greek yogurt 150 g**
- **Sugar 120 g**
- **Eggs (about 4) 220 g**
- **Baking powder for sweets 16 g**
- **Lemon zest 1**

Start by pouring the eggs into a large bowl and start whipping them with forks or with an electric whisk, then add the sugar little by little continuing to work for about 5 minutes. Add the yogurt and mix it again with the whisk. Sift the yeast and flour into a separate bowl and add them a spoon at a time, keeping the whisk in action. Finally, add the grated lemon zest and mix again. Now wash the apples, cut them into wedges, and remove the peel. Cut the wedges into cubes and add them to the dough, then mix with a spatula to incorporate them evenly. Line a muffin pan with paper cups and fill them with about two tablespoons of dough each. Bake in a preheated static oven at 180 ° for about 25-28 minutes. Once cooked, take it out of the oven and let it cool. Your apple muffins are ready to taste!

8) Baked Frittata

Ingredients:

- **Eggs 8**
- **Grated cheese 100 g**
- **Chives to taste**
- **Thyme to taste**
- **Salt to taste**
- **Extra virgin olive oil 10 g**

FOR BRUSHING AND SPREADING THE TRAY

- **Extra virgin olive oil to taste**
- **Breadcrumbs to taste**

To prepare the frittata, start by oiling a 26x19 cm rectangular baking dish, then line it with breadcrumbs 2. Beat the eggs, add the grated cheese, oil, finely chopped chives. Continue with peeled thyme, salt. Then keep on beating for a few moments until a homogeneous mixture is obtained. Transfer everything to the oven dish and cook in a preheated static oven at 170 ° for 25 minutes. Once ready, serve your frittata in the hot oven to start the day!

9) Porridge

Ingredients:

- **Oat flakes 140 g**
- **Skimmed milk 220 g220 g**
- **Water 200 g**
- **Salt to taste**

TO SEAL
- **Honey to taste**
- **Strawberries to taste**
- **Flaked almonds to taste**

To make the porridge first, pour the oats into a bowl, cover with water and leave to soak for about an hour, (it is preferable to leave it to soak the night before). Pour the oats into the saucepan, add the milk, add a pinch of salt and cook the mixture for about 4-5 minutes, stirring often. When the oats are soft and have absorbed the milk, turn off the heat and transfer the porridge to a bowl and flavor with the honey. Garnish with slices of fresh strawberries and almonds. Serve your lukewarm porridge.

10) Salted Plumcake

Ingredients:
- **Corn flour 200 g**
- **Eggs 3**
- **Raw ham 150 g**
- **Skimmed milk 150 ml**
- **Extra virgin olive oil 60 ml**
- **Salt to taste**
- **Instant yeast for savory preparations 1 sachet**
- **Grated cheese 150 g**

To prepare the salted plumcake, start by sifting the yeast and flour in a bowl, then add the grated cheese. Mix the ingredients well and stir in the raw ham, mix again. Then add the extra virgin olive oil flush. In another bowl, beat the eggs with the milk and salt and add the liquid, thus obtained to the mixture of flour, cheese, and ham. Stir with a spoon until the ingredients are well mixed. Grease and flour a plumcake mold with a capacity of one liter and put the dough inside. Level it with the back of a spoon and bake in a preheated oven at 180 ° C for 45/50 minutes, doing a toothpick test to check its cooking. When the salted plumcake is cooked, wait until it is warm before removing it from the mold, then let it cool completely. Serve your salted plumcake!

Chapter 4: Recipes for starter

1) Boiled eggs

Ingredients:

- **4 fresh eggs**

To prepare the hard-boiled eggs, start by placing the whole eggs in a large saucepan and pour the cold water (the water will have to cover the eggs). Then put the saucepan on the fire and let it boil. From the boil, calculate 9 minutes of cooking. After 9 minutes, remove the saucepan from the heat and pass it under fresh running water to cool the eggs. This will allow you to peel them without getting burned; carefully remove all the shells, then divide the eggs in half, and you will discover the perfectly cooked interior! Boiled eggs are ready to be eaten as you like!

2) Gratinated prawns

Ingredients:

- **Gratinated prawns**
- **Shrimp (about 16) 200 g**
- **Salt to taste**
- **White wine 80 ml**

FOR THE PANURE
- **Breadcrumbs 50 g**
- **Parmesan 25 g**
- **Extra virgin olive oil to taste**
- **Parsley to be chopped 10 g**
- **Salt to taste**

We start cleaning the shellfish by peeling them and leaving the tail, cut the back of the shrimp with a knife to eliminate the black thread inside.

Place two prawns in each shell (or in any container of your imagination), to occupy the interior, and pour a spoonful of white wine into each one, directly on the prawns. To prepare the panure: in a bowl, arrange the breadcrumbs, the chopped parsley, the grated Parmesan, and the salt. Pour a drizzle of oil and mix.

Cover the shells with a few tablespoons of panure and add a drizzle of oil. Arrange the shells with the prawns on a baking tray covered with parchment paper and bake at 180 degrees for about 25 minutes. Now you are ready to serve this imaginative dish!

3) Pineapple stuffed with shrimp

Ingredients:

- **Pineapple of about 1 kg 1**
- **Shrimp 450 g**
- **Chives 6 strands**
- **Mint 5 leaves**
- **Extra virgin olive oil to taste**
- **Salt to taste**
- **Mixed salad**

Let's start by cleaning the shrimp (you can also use the frozen ones), eliminating the fillet inside. Rinse them under running water, then lift your head with your hands and lift your legs. At this point, shell them. Once all the prawns have been cleaned, pour a drizzle of oil into a large pan. Add the peeled shrimp to the pan and brown them on both sides. Then turn off the heat and put them in a small bowl to cool them. Prepare the pineapple that will be the salad's container: choose a ripe pineapple and divide it in half. Cut the inner pulp along the perimeter of both halves to extract all the pulp without breaking it. Eliminate the most callused part of the pulp. From the extracted pulp, obtain medium-sized pineapple cubes to add to the salad. Now chop the aromas: chives and mint. Take the mixed salad previously washed under water and pour it into the pineapple container along with its cubes. Also, add the previously sautéed prawns. Then add the aromatic herbs to the salad: chives, minced mint salt, a drizzle of oil, and mix the ingredients to blend the flavors. Now that the salad is ready, you can start stuffing the pineapple until it is full. Now you can serve your pineapple shrimp salad for a beautiful and fresh summer lunch!

4) Chickpea shrimp and arugula salad

Ingredients:

- **Shrimp 1 kg**
- **Pre-cooked chickpeas 240 g**
- **Rocket 150 g**
- **Pine nuts 30 g**
- **TO CONDITION**

- **Lemon juice 1**
- **Extra virgin olive oil to taste**
- **Salt to taste**

To make the chickpea shrimp and rocket salad, start by cleaning the shrimp (or prawns) by removing the head, the carapace, and the intestines inside. Now toast the pine nuts in a pan for 4-5 minutes until they are browned and set aside. Heat a drizzle of oil in a pan, put the prawns, salt, use a pinch of pepper. Cook them on high heat for 5 -6 minutes. Once cooked, transfer them to a small bowl to cool.

Now drain the pre-cooked chickpeas (you can also use the dried ones but keep them soak and cook them for at least three hours so they will be ready for preparation). In the same pan used for the prawns, heat the chickpeas so that they take on the flavor of the shellfish. Now that all the ingredients are ready, you can compose the salad: In a large bowl, put the washed and dried arugula.

Add the prawns, chickpeas and toasted pine nuts and mix everything together. Finally, take care of the dressing: prepare an emulsion with oil, salt, and the juice of half a lemon. Season the salad with the prepared dressing. Your chickpea shrimp and rocket salad are now ready!

5) Vegetable crudités

Ingredients:

- **Celery 2**
- **Carrots 2**
- **Fennel 1**
- **Yellow peppers 1/2**
- **1/2 red peppers**
- **Chicory 1**
- **Radishes 12**
- **Extra virgin olive oil to taste**
- **Lemon juice to taste**
- **Salt to taste**

Take two stalks of tender celery and clean them by removing the leaves and any filaments. Cut the stalks into two parts of equal length and then cut the sticks by cutting the pieces obtained for the length. Take the fennel, remove the ends with the leaves, and then also the opposite one; now cut the fennel into four equal parts, which you will reduce again in half.

Take the half peppers, remove the filaments and the internal white parts, then cut the peppers into strips. Remove the radish leaves and wash the radishes under running water.

Peel the carrots, tick the ends, and cut them into parallel slices, which you will then divide into sticks. Remove the outer leaves of the radicchio and keep them fresh and intact by detaching them from its base. Now put the vegetables cut into small glasses and prepare bowls containing extra virgin olive oil. To prepare the sauce, mix together in a salt oil container, lemon, and beat vigorously with a fork to emulsify everything or do it with an immersion blender. Serve your vegetable sticks accompanied by the sauce.

6) Chunks of quinoa

Ingredients:

- **Quinoa 150 g**
- **Small zucchini 2**
- **Eggs 1**
- **Grated cheese 50 g**
- **Grated lemon zest 1**
- **Fresh ginger to be grated to taste**
- **Salt to taste**

Proceed by draining the quinoa and passing it under cold water to stop cooking. At this point, wash the zucchini and peel them, then peel and peel the fresh ginger. Grate the zucchini and place them in a large bowl, where you will add the grated fresh ginger and the grated lemon zest.

Add the boiled quinoa to the grated zucchini, ginger, and lemon zest and add the grated cheese and egg. Season with salt and mix the ingredients until you obtain a homogeneous mixture. Now put the mixture in baking molds (you can also use a non-stick muffin mold) and place them on a baking sheet. Compact the mixture inside the shapes with the help of the back of a spoon, in order to better define the shape of the morsels. Now bake them in an oven already preheated in static mode at 180 ° for 25 minutes (if you use a fan oven cook them at 160 ° for 20 minutes), until the surface is golden brown. At this point, the quinoa morsels are ready to be tasted!

7) Eggplant Caviar

Ingredients:

- **Eggplant (about 3) 1 kg**
- **½ lemon juice**
- **Mint 4 leaves**
- **Extra virgin olive oil 2 tbsp**
- **Salt to taste**

Wash the eggplant, then dry them. Arrange them on a dripping pan lined with a sheet of parchment paper. Cook them in a preheated static oven at 180 ° for at least 60 minutes (or at 160 ° for 50 minutes if in a fan oven).

Now remove the eggplants from the oven, and with a knife, remove the peel and with a spoon take the pulp contained inside. Put the pulp in a narrow mesh strainer and with the

back of a spoon press it, so that it releases the excess liquid. Put the pulp in a mixer equipped with blades and add the oil.

Season with salt and add the mint after which operate the blades until you get a thick and homogeneous puree. Transfer everything to a small bowl, then squeeze the juice of half a lemon into the puree you have obtained. Mix everything, and your eggplant caviar is ready to be served.

8) Octopus salad

Ingredients:

- **Octopus to clean 1 kg**
- **Carrots 1**
- **Celery 1 rib**
- **Laurel 2 leaves**
- **Salt up to 4 g**

TO CONDITION
- **Parsley 10 g**
- **Lemon juice 10 g**
- **Extra virgin olive oil 30 g**
- **Black pepper 1 pinch**
- **Salt up to a pinch**

Start with the octopus, rinse it under running water, with a knife cut the bag at eye level to eliminate them, then also remove the beak. Rinse the octopus again under running water and remove the entrails from the bag by washing it carefully inside (You can also use the frozen one). Peel the carrot, then cut it into coarse pieces.

Do the same thing with celery. Place a large saucepan with water on the fire, pour the coast of celery into pieces, the pieces of carrot, the bay leaves, and add the salt. When the water has touched the boil, dip the octopus in the pan and cook over very low heat for 40-45 minutes, covering with a lid. As it cooks, you can remove residues and foam that are created on the surface from the water. At the end of the cooking, let the octopus cool in the same water so that it is soft. Transfer it to the cutting board and, with a knife, separate the head from the tentacles and divide them in half. Cut the tentacles into small pieces. Cut the head into small pieces and pour everything into a bowl. For the dressing, squeeze the lemon, then wash and finely chop the parsley. Make the dressing by pouring the juice, parsley, lemon juice, oil, and salt into a jar. Close and mix. Pour the mixture over the octopus, mix well, and serve your octopus salad!

9) Marinated anchovies

Ingredients:

- **Anchovies (chopped) 500 g**
- **Lemon juice 150 g**
- **Parsley 20 g**
- **Extra virgin olive oil 140 g**
- **Fine salt**

To prepare the marinated anchovies started with the marinade: pour the parsley together with 40 g of olive oil in a mixer and chop everything for a few moments. Squeeze the lemons, and collect the juice in a container together with the olive oil and season with salt. Mix well and when the two compounds have bonded together, add the chopped parsley.

Keep stirring and keep the marinade aside. Meanwhile, move on to cleaning the anchovies; given that they will not undergo cooking, it is important to make sure that they were cut down during the purchase phase (always choose fresh anchovies to buy in your trusted fish shop); for greater safety, it is recommended to freeze for at least 96 hours at -18 degrees (already gutted) and then thaw to use in the recipe.

 Then take off the head, then pull away the central bone and the entrails, finally rinse the fillets underwater, taking care not to divide the fish into two halves. Place the well-cleaned anchovy fillets side by side in a large container and pour the marinade you have prepared, then cover with plastic wrap. Let stand for at least 5 hours at room temperature.

After the necessary time, remove the film, and finally drain them slightly from the marinade and arrange the marinated anchovies on a plate to serve and enjoy them as an appetizer!

10) Eggplant and tofu meatballs

Ingredients:
- **100 g of tofu**
- **1 large eggplant**
- **1 clove of garlic**
- **2 sprigs of parsley**
- **1 tablespoon of flour**
- **4 tablespoons of breadcrumbs**
- **salt**
- **oil to taste**

Cook the whole eggplant in the oven; once cooked, sauté its pulp in a pan in a garlic sauce. Season with salt and add the crumbled tofu. Mix the ingredients, if necessary, with a little flour. Complete the preparation with chopped parsley. Prepare meatballs the size of an apricot, dip them in breadcrumbs, bake them or fry them in a pan, according to preference.

Chapter 5: First dishes

1) Risotto with chickpeas

Ingredients:

- **140 grams of brown rice**
- **200 grams of boiled chickpeas**
- **1 carrot**
- **1 teaspoon of extra virgin olive oil**
- **vegetable broth**

Sauté the carrot cut into small pieces with the oil in a pan. Mix and combine 150 grams of boiled chickpeas, giving flavor to everything. Add the rice and continue cooking for 15 minutes or as long as the packaging. Occasionally pour a ladle of vegetable rice broth if you see that the bottom of the pan is dry and without liquid. Cook the rice completely, and at the end of the cooking, add the remaining chickpeas. Your risotto is ready to be eaten!

2) Barley and bean soup

Ingredients:
- **200 g of cooked beans**
- **150 g of pearl barley**
- **1 small carrot**
- **1 stalk of celery**
- **100 g approx. of pumpkin pulp**
- **1 sprig of parsley**
- **1 clove of garlic**
- **4 tablespoons of oil**
- **1 pinch of chilli**
- **salt**

Boil the barley in 400 ml of water with a pinch of salt, for about 40 minutes, in a covered pot. Prepare a mixture of garlic, celery, carrot, and parsley; cut the pumpkin into cubes. Fry the mixture in oil in a large pot with a pinch of salt; then add the pumpkin and let it simmer for five minutes, until softened, possibly with a little water. Then add the barley and beans with their cooking water or a little broth to get the right consistency (the soup should be creamy); bring to a boil and cook for another 5 minutes. Season with a pinch of chili and serve hot. Alternatively, you can cook the barley directly with the vegetables and add the beans towards cooking.

3) Pasta and zucchini

Ingredients:

- **Pasta 320 g**
- **Zucchini 650 g**
- **Basil to taste**
- **Salt to taste**
- **Extra virgin olive oil 20 g**
- **Black pepper to taste**
- **Garlic 1 clove**

To prepare pasta and zucchini, boil the water in a large saucepan and salt when it has come to a boil. In the meantime, wash and dry the zucchini, cut them into cubes or slices. In a large enough pan, pour the extra virgin olive oil and heat it over low heat together with a whole clove of garlic already peeled.

As soon as the oil is hot, add the zucchini, add salt and pepper and cook for 5-6 minutes, stirring occasionally, then remove the garlic. In the meantime, boil the pasta in boiling salted water and drain it al dente, keeping some cooking water aside.

Pour the pasta into the pan with the zucchini, together with a little cooking water, sauté the pasta, stir and then turn off. Perfume everything with a little chopped basil by hand, and your pasta and zucchini are ready to be enjoyed.

Before bringing to the table, remove the bay leaves and possibly also the cloves and serve hot.

4)   Cream of spinach with pine nuts

Ingredients:
- **1 kg of spinach**
- **2 shallots**
- **500 ml of vegetable broth**
- **100 ml of soy milk**
- **100 g of tofu**
- **2 tablespoons of flour**
- **2 tablespoons of pine nuts**
- **2 teaspoons of turmeric**
- **2 tablespoons of oil**
- **salt and pepper**

Clean the spinach, wash and drain them. Finely chop the shallots and let them soften in a saucepan with a little broth for about ten minutes. Add the flour, stir so that it does not form lumps, and add the spinach. Add salt, stir briefly and pour in the warmed milk and remaining broth, tofu, and turmeric. Cook for about ten minutes and blend by immersion. Peppered, seasoned with oil, and served garnished with lightly toasted pine nuts and, if desired, with oatcakes

5) Indian rice

Ingredients:
- **300 g of wholemeal basmati rice**
- **1 carrot**
- **200 g of peas**
- **2 shallots**
- **1 piece of cinnamon**
- **2 cardamom capsules**
- **1 heaped teaspoon of turmeric**
- **1 clove**
- **1 bay leaf**
- **1 tablespoon of raisins**
- **20 almonds**
- **3 tablespoons of oil**
- **salt and pepper**

Put the rice in a saucepan, cover it with 800 ml of water, close with the lid, and boil. Turn down the heat. Rinse the raisins and soak them in warm water for about ten minutes. Put the chopped shallots in a pan with the cinnamon, the cardamom seeds, the turmeric, the clove, and the bay leaf. Add the soaking water from the raisins and let it soften over medium heat, stirring often. Transfer to the saucepan with the rice. When 30 minutes have passed, add the peas, raisins, and carrot cut into cubes. Cook for another 15-20 minutes until the liquid has run out. Remove the bay leaf, the carnation, and the cinnamon. Season with salt, season with oil and pepper. Complete with the sliced almonds and serve.

6) Rice and zucchini croquettes with saffron sauce

Ingredients:
For the croquettes:
- 350 g of brown rice
- 850 ml of water
- 800 g of zucchini
- 2 tablespoons of oil
- 1 teaspoon of salt
- 1 bunch of parsley
- 1 clove of garlic
- salt and pepper

For the saffron sauce:
- 250 ml of soy milk
- 30 ml of oil
- 30 g of rice flour
- 1 sachet of saffron and salt

Sauté the chopped garlic and parsley in a little oil. Add and stew the sliced zucchini with salt and pepper for 10 minutes. Puree about 1/3 of the zucchini. Wash the rice, drain it and cook it in salted water, covered and without stirring, for about 35 minutes. Season the rice with the salt and the zucchini not passed, stir and continue cooking for another 5 minutes. Let it cool (if it is too soft, let it cool completely or add some breadcrumbs), then form some meatballs that you will bake in the oven at 200 ° for about 15-20 minutes. To prepare the sauce, brown the flour in a saucepan with the oil, then add the milk. Bring to a boil and let it thicken over low heat, stirring with a whisk. Salt and add the saffron and the zucchini puree.

7) Broccoli and sweet potato pie

Ingredients:
- **300 g of sweet potatoes**
- **400 g of broccoli**
- **2 cloves of garlic**
- **1 bunch of parsley**
- **1 glass of vegetable broth**
- **3 tablespoons of oil**
- **salt**

Peel and wash the sweet potatoes, then cut them into slices that are not too thick. Peel and clean the broccoli; slice the stems and divide the flowers into florets. Finely chop garlic and parsley. Line a baking sheet with parchment paper and brush it with a tablespoon of oil mixed with water. Make the first layer with the potatoes and a pinch of salt, a second with the broccoli and a little more salt, a third with garlic and parsley. Finish with the potatoes and pour over all the broth. Bake at 190 degrees for about 40 minutes. When cooked, season with the remaining oil and serve.

8) Spelled and leek lasagna

Ingredients:
- **300 g of lasagne**
- **2 leeks**
- **250 g of mozzarella**
- **70 g of parmesan cheese**
- **extra virgin olive oil**
- **½ glass of milk**

Clean the leeks, cut them lengthwise, and soak them in freshwater for about 30 minutes. Meanwhile, in a full pot of boiling water, cook the lasagna for about 5 minutes and set it aside. Drain the leeks and put them to stew in a pan with a drizzle of oil without adding salt because they are already delicious. Cook them for about twenty minutes. Take a pan, preferably rectangular, and form the layers: start by placing a layer of pasta on the pan's bottom and lay the leeks on top. Take the mozzarella, cut it into small pieces, and put them on top of the leeks. Finish with a sprinkling of parmesan cheese. Continue to alternate puff pastry, leek, mozzarella, and parmesan, until all the ingredients are used up. Once the last sheet is finished, pour the milk over the lasagna and complete it with a shower of parmesan cheese. Bake for 25 minutes at 180 °.

9)   Spaghetti in tofu cream with spinach and hazelnuts

Ingredients:
- **350 g of wholemeal spaghetti**
- **200 g of fresh spinach**
- **80 g of hazelnuts**

For the olive tofu cream
- **200 g of natural tofu**
- **the juice of half a lemon**
- **1 cup of capers**
- **1 cup of olives**
- **a large tuft of chopped parsley**
- **3 tablespoons of olive oil**
- **a tablespoon of soy sauce**
- **a pinch of salt**
- **1 small clove of garlic**

Put the water on the fire to cook the pasta; once it reaches a boil, add salt and throw the wholemeal spaghetti. In the meantime, take a saucepan with a little water and put it on the stove: as soon as it boils, add a pinch of salt and dip the natural tofu block cut into small pieces. Boil for a minute, drain, and put it in the blender, where you will add the olives without the stones, the sprig of parsley, the capers, the juice of half a lemon, the clove of garlic, the oil, the soy sauce, and the pinch of salt. To soften, you can add a few tablespoons of the tofu boiling water. Blend until you get a soft and homogeneous cream that you will keep aside. Then wash the fresh spinach leaves; you can roughly cut them or leave them whole. Dry them and keep them aside. Then take a non-stick pan and toast the hazelnuts, coarsely chopped. Drain the pasta and put it in a large bowl, and add the tofu cream to the olives; if necessary, help yourself with a little tofu cooking water, as above. Add the fresh spinach leaves, toasted hazelnuts, and finally a drizzle of raw oil. If you wish, you can also add a splash of fresh oregano or paprika powder. Serve the spaghetti hot and steaming. Simple and tasty!

8) Rice cake

Ingredients:

- Champignon mushrooms 500 g

- Rice 300 g

- Grated cheese 150 g

- Vegetable broth about 750 ml

- 1 sprig parsley

- Salt to taste

Dedicate yourself to the champignon mushrooms, wash and peel them, then remove the part of the stem with the roots and cut the head of the champignons into rather thin slices. Chop the fresh parsley. In a large pan pour a drizzle of oil then add the champignon mushrooms and chopped parsley. Fry over low heat for about 3 minutes. Stir and cook the mushrooms for about 5 minutes. Season with salt and then cook for about 10 minutes over moderate heat. The mushrooms will not have to cook completely because they will then finish cooking in the oven. While the mushrooms are cooking, pour the oil into a large pan, pour in the rice, brown for a couple of minutes, stirring with a wooden spoon.

Continue cooking the risotto for about 20 minutes, adding the vegetable broth a little at a time with a ladle when you see that the rice is devoid of liquid. When the rice is cooked for 2 minutes, pour in the grated cheese, stir, turn off the heat and let the risotto rest for a few minutes. Take a baking tray and cover it with parchment paper. Then with a spoon start creating a layer of rice, compacting it with the back of the spoon.When you have covered the bottom, create a layer of mushrooms, then rice, so that the result is two layers with the mushroom filling. Finally, sprinkle the top with the leftover cheese. Finally bake in a preheated static oven at 200 ° for about 30 minutes (if oven at 180 ° for about 25 minutes). Then remove from the oven and let it cool.

Chapter 6: Main courses

1) Veal roast, apples and potatoes

Ingredients:

- **600 grams of veal fillet**
- **1 teaspoon of oil**
- **2 sprigs of rosemary**
- **half a glass of white wine**
- **2 apples**
- **250 grams of potatoes**
- **Salt**

Put the meat in a pan with oil, rosemary, and a pinch of salt. Brown it by blending with the white wine. Combine the apples with the peel and the chopped potatoes. Bake at 200 degrees for about 30 minutes. Get out of the oven, remove the meat, and let it cool. Cut it into slices and serve with potatoes and apples.

2) Poached eggs

Ingredients:

- **Very fresh, organic eggs 4**
- **Coarse salt to taste**
- **White wine vinegar 10 g**
- **TO ACCOMPANY**
- **4 slices bread**

When the salt has dissolved, and the water starts to boil lightly (it must not boil strongly), lower the flame and with a whisk stir always in the same direction to create a vortex in the water; then break an egg into a small bowl and pour it in the center of the vortex. Cook the egg like this for 2 minutes. Do not mix or move the egg. Drain the egg with the help of a slotted spoon, then lay it on the toasted bread and serve your hot poached eggs.

3) Crispy salmon

Ingredients:
- **Salmon fillet (4 of 250 g each) 1 kg**
- **Bread 100 g**
- **1 sprig parsley**
- **Thyme 4 sprigs**
- **Rosemary 2 sprigs**
- **Lemon zest 1**
- **Extra virgin olive oil 50 g**
- **White pepper in grains 1 tsp**
- **Salt up to taste**

First, prepare the breading: cut the bread into pieces and put it in a mixer, the peeled thyme, the needles of rosemary and parsley. Pour in the oil too, then add the lemon zest, salt and white pepper. Blend until you get a coarse consistency. Now take care of the salmon fillets: remove the skin with a thin-bladed knife and remove the bones with the help of a kitchen tongs, then transfer the fillets to a drip pan lined with parchment paper and cover them with the breading, making it adhere well with your hands. . After covering the fillets evenly, cook in a preheated convection oven at 190 ° for about 20 minutes. After the cooking time, take out and serve your crispy salmon hot!

4) Sea bass with herb in salt crust

Ingredients:

- **Salt up to 1 kg**
- **Sea bass 800 g**
- **Coarse salt 1 kg**
- **Sage 6 leaves**
- **Thyme 6 sprigs**
- **Parsley 1 bunch**
- **Laurel 4 leaves**
- **Rosemary 3 sprigs**
- **Garlic 1 clove**
- **Lemons 1**

Spread a sheet of parchment paper on a baking sheet and then lay a thin layer (about 1.5 cm) of the mixture obtained, which will form the cooking bed for the sea bass. Now place the sea bass on the bed of salt that you previously flavored by placing it in your belly aromatic herbs, minced garlic, and lemon zest; now cover the sea bass with the salt mixture by pressing it gently to make the dough adhere well and give a shape that adheres to the fish 11. Bake for about 40 minutes (if instead of 1-kilo sea bass, you have taken a smaller one 400 / About 500gr the cooking time will be about 25-30 minutes). After 40 minutes, remove the sea bass from the oven, let it rest for a few moments, then, using a small hammer, break the salt crust and proceed to remove the skin of the fish. Open it in two by removing the central bone, as in any other oven preparation. You can accompany the sea bass, with boiled potatoes, or also cooked in the oven. Season with a drizzle of extra virgin olive oil, not to cover the aroma and delicate flavor of the sea bass.

5) Chicken and zucchini salad

Ingredients:

- **Sliced chicken breast 400 g**
- **Zucchini 200 g**
- **Eggplants 200 g**
- **Mixed salad 60 g**
- **Salt to taste**
- **Extra virgin olive oil to taste**
-

FOR MARINATING

- **Extra virgin olive oil 25 g**
- **Wildflower honey 25 g**
- **½ lemon juice**
- **Thyme to taste**
- **Salt to taste**

To prepare the chicken and zucchini salad, we must first marinate the chicken. Arrange the chicken breasts in an ovenproof dish, pour the oil inside, season with salt, the juice of half a lemon, honey, and a few sprigs of thyme. Turn the slices over both so that the entire surface of the meat is well marinated, then cover the baking dish with plastic wrap and let it sit for one hour at room temperature. Now move on to the preparation of the vegetables. Wash the zucchini, cut the ends, and cut them lengthwise with a sliced knife about 1 cm thick. Do the same thing with eggplants too. Now heat the grill, grease it with a drizzle of oil, then lay the slices of zucchini and grill them on both sides, then salt. Also, grill and salt the eggplants, turning them on both sides, then switch to the chicken, which you will pick from the marinade to put it on the grill. Once grilled, cut the eggplants, zucchini, and chicken slices into strips about 2 cm long. Let the grilled vegetables cool, and transfer them to a bowl with the chicken and the mixed salad, then mix and transfer to the dishes. The chicken and zucchini salad are ready to be served!

6) Pan-fried sea bream

Ingredients:

- **Sea bream (2 pieces) 1100 g**

- **Extra virgin olive oil 30 g**

- **Carrots 150 g**

- **Zucchini150 g**

- **Garlic 1 clove**

- **Thyme to taste**

To prepare the sea bream in a pan, first of all, you have to clean the fish (otherwise you can buy it already gutted). Make a cut on the belly with scissors and remove the entrails with your hands, then rinse the inside thoroughly under water and eliminate the scales using a blade of a knife; do this under running water so as not to spread the scales around. Now let's cut the vegetables: wash and peel the carrots, then cut the ends and cut them into rounds. Wash and peel the courgettes and cut them into cubes. Pour the oil into a large non-stick pan, add a clove of poached garlic and fry it for a couple of minutes. When the oil is flavored, remove the garlic from the pan and lay the sea bream inside, then add the zucchini, carrots, and thyme sprigs and salt to taste. Cover the pan with a lid and cook over medium heat for 7 minutes, then turn the sea bream with the help of 2 spatulas being careful not to break them; cover again with the lid and cook for another 7 minutes. Cooking times may vary depending on the weight of the sea bream you will use. Pan-fried sea bream is ready to eat!

7) Cod medallions and broccoli

Ingredients:

- **Cod fillet 400 g**
- **Broccoli 200 g**
- **Potatoes 400 g**
- **Marjoram 3 sprigs**
- **Extra virgin olive oil to taste**
- **Salt to taste**

To prepare the medallions of cod and broccoli, first, we take the cod fillets (they should also be frozen well, in that case, let them thaw for at least 2-3 hours before). Then put two saucepans on the fire with water to bring to a boil; in one dip the potatoes, calculate them 30-40 minutes. The time may vary depending on the size of the potatoes, so remember to check the degree of cooking with a fork.

If the fork easily penetrates inside the potatoes, it means it is cooked. In the meantime, wash the broccoli, put them in the other pan, and when the water boils boil them for about 5 minutes. After 5 minutes, drain the broccoli and coarsely chop them, then let them cool. When the potatoes are ready, peel and mash them with a potato masher in a large bowl, then preheat the oven to 200 ° in static mode. Finally, take the cod fillets and cut them into several, not too small parts. When the vegetables have cooled, take the bowl where you have mashed the potatoes, add the chopped broccoli and cod, salt and add the marjoram leaves, then knead with your hands to mix all the ingredients. Take some dough and shape it with a pastry cutter to form the medallions. Place the medallions on a dripping pan lined with parchment paper, season with a little oil, then cook in a preheated static oven at 200 ° for about 20 minutes.

After the cooking time of the medallions, take them out of the oven and transfer them to a serving dish; add a few leaves of marjoram and season with a drizzle of raw oil. Your cod and broccoli medallions are ready to be brought to the table!

8) Baked chicken legs

Ingredients:

- **Chicken legs 4**
- **Potatoes 500 g**
- **Salt to taste**
- **Extra virgin olive oil 50 g**
- **Rosemary 3 sprigs**
- **Thyme 3 sprigs**

Put the chicken legs in a baking dish and season with salt, oil, and marinate. Peel the potatoes, cut them into wedges, and transfer them into a dripping pan lined with parchment paper. Season with salt, oil (optional pepper but do not overdo it), then add the chicken legs and flavor everything with the sprigs of thyme and rosemary. Bake in a preheated static oven at 180 ° for 80 minutes, turning them halfway through cooking. When they are golden brown, take them out of the oven and serve them!

9) Roasted rabbit

Ingredients:

- **Rabbit in pieces 1.2 kg**
- **4 sprigs rosemary**
- **Salt to taste**
- **Vegetable broth 150 g**
- **Potatoes 800 g**
- **Thyme 4 sprigs**
- **White wine 40 g**
- **Bay leaf 1 leaf**
- **Extra virgin olive oil 70 g**

To prepare the rabbit in the oven, start by preparing the vegetable broth a couple of hours before, chop the rosemary, then transfer half of it to a pan where you have poured 40 g of oil.

Add a bay leaf and let it cook over low heat for 2-3 minutes. At this point, raise the heat and add the rabbit pieces, brown them on both sides for 3-4 minutes, add salt and deglaze with the white wine. Once the alcoholic phase has evaporated, add a ladle of broth and cook over low heat for another 5-6 minutes.

Meanwhile, prepare the potatoes, peel them, cut them into large enough pieces, and transfer them to a bowl. Add chopped rosemary, thyme leaves and salt to the potatoes. Sprinkle with 20 g of oil and mix. Transfer everything to a large pan, oiled with about 10 g of oil. Then arrange the browned rabbit pieces as well. Add the remaining vegetable broth and cook the rabbit together with the potatoes in a preheated static oven at 200 ° for 40 minutes. Once cooked, serve your rabbit in the oven

10) Salad baskets with turkey

Ingredients:
- **Turkey breast 250 g**
- **Baby lettuce 100 g**
- **Cashews 25 g**
- **Carrots 1**
- **Parsley to taste**
- **Extra virgin olive oil q.s.**

Place the turkey breast on a cutting board and cut it into irregular pieces. Then take a non-stick pan, heat a drizzle of oil. Add the turkey breast bites and salt. Cook the morsels for about 10 minutes, turning them from time to time to cook them inside until they are golden brown. When the turkey morsels are cooked, transfer them to a mixer, operate for a few seconds until the meat is well chopped, and then transfer the blended mixture into a large bowl. At this point, place the cashews on a cutting board and chop them coarsely. Sauté the chopped cashews in a non-stick pan and toast them for a few minutes, until crisp and darker. Then add the toasted cashews to the chopped turkey bites. Then take a carrot, peel it and divide it in half. After that, slice it into tiny cubes. Also, wash the parsley under running water and chop finely on a cutting board. At this point, add the diced carrot and chopped parsley to the mixture. Now wash the salad carefully and leaf it through, placing the crispest and most curved leaves on a serving dish. Then proceed to fill them with the dough. Your baskets of lettuce with turkey are ready to be served.

Chapter 7: Recipes for Side dish

1) Fennel in a pan

Ingredients:

- **Fennel (about 2) 900 g**
- **Extra virgin olive oil 15 g**
- **Himalayan salt (pink) to taste**
- **Marjoram to taste**
- **Thyme to taste**

To make the fennel in a pan, start by washing the fennel, then clean them by cutting the base of the core, and the stalks, after which cut them into wedges.

Once the fennel is cut, you can proceed with cooking: heat the extra virgin olive oil in a pan, then add the fennel wedges and cook for about 5 minutes on high heat. Season with the Himalayan salt and season with the leaves of marjoram and thyme. Continue cooking for another 5 minutes to keep the fennel crunchy otherwise, and you can continue cooking them for a few more minutes if you like them softer. Serve your fennel hot in a pan.

2) Carrot and sweet potato roll with millet

Ingredients:
- **200 g of carrots**
- **1 sweet potato**
- **1 tablespoon of corn starch**
- **200 g of cooked millet**
- **3 tablespoons of oil**
- **salt**

To garnish
- **100 g of peeled pumpkin**
- **a few leaves of salad**
- **1 tablespoon of oil**
- **salt**

Clean the carrots and the potato, chop them and steam them for about 10 minutes. Let them cool, then blend them in the mixer with the millet, starch, oil, and salt. Remove the salami mixture and wrap it in cotton gauze, closing them like candy with a piece of string. Steam them for 15-20 minutes. Wait until they are completely cold and cut them into slices. Wash the salad, dry it and cut it into strips; coarsely grate the pumpkin. Arrange the rolls on a serving dish, surround them with the prepared garnish seasoned with oil and salt.

3) Grilled vegetables

Ingredients:

- **Zucchini 300 g**
- **Eggplants 450 g**
- **Peppers 850 g**
- **Salt to taste**

To prepare the grilled vegetables, wash all the vegetables under running fresh water, and dry them. Cut the zucchini and eggplants into slices; take the peppers, remove the upper part, divide them in half, and with a knife remove the white filaments and the seeds that are inside. Cut them into rather large cubes and set aside. Cut all the vegetables, heat the grill.

When the grill is hot, cook the vegetables a little at a time. Spread the peppers close to each other, grilling them for 5 minutes and turning them over for even cooking, then put the eggplants on the fire for 3 minutes and continue with the zucchini for another 3 minutes. Remember to always turn the vegetables over for even cooking. Finally, season the grilled vegetables with olive oil and salt.

4) Mashed potatoes

Ingredients:

- Yellow potatoes 1 kg

- Whole skimmed 200 g

- Light butter 30 g

- Parmigiano Reggiano to be grated 30 g

- Salt to taste

- Nutmeg to taste

Let's start by boiling the potatoes. Then pour them in a large pot and cover with plenty of water. Put the pan on the fire, and when the water has boiled, it will take 40 to 50 minutes. The cooking times depend on the size of the potatoes. Reached the 40 minutes of cooking skewer a potato with a fork and see if it penetrates easily; at that point, it is cooked. Drain and let it cool for a few minutes because you will have to take advantage that the potatoes are still very hot to peel them easily.

After peeling the potatoes, pour them into the potato masher, pour them directly into the cooking pan. Then add a pinch of salt and flavor by grating a little nutmeg. In the meantime, put the milk in a saucepan.

Meanwhile, light over a low flame where there is a pot with the mashed potatoes, and when the milk is hot, pour it inside and mix with a whisk until the mixture is well blended. Then turn off the heat and stir adding butter and Parmesan cheese. Your mashed potato is read.

5) Baked au gratin vegetables

Ingredients:

- Zucchini 300 g
- Eggplants 180 g long
- Red peppers 250 g
- Yellow peppers 250 g
- Extra virgin olive oil 20 g
- Salt to taste

FOR BREADING

- Breadcrumbs 30 g
- Parmesan cheese DOP to be grated 30 g
- Dried oregano to taste

First, cut the vegetables: wash the eggplants, remove the ends, and cut them diagonally into slices 2-3 cm thick; do the same thing with the zucchini. Finally, wash the peppers, empty them of the seeds and internal filaments and cut them first in half and then into pieces more or less as big as the slices of eggplants and zucchini.

Arrange the cut vegetables in a pan lined with parchment paper, then season with salt and olive oil 6. Bake the pan in a static preheated oven at 180 ° for 45 minutes. In the meantime, prepare the breadcrumbs for the vegetables: In a bowl, add the breadcrumbs with the grated Parmesan and the oregano, and mix well.

After 45 minutes, remove the vegetables from the oven, spread the breadcrumbs over all the vegetables with a spoon. Bake at 180 ° again for another 15 minutes. Your side dish is ready!

6) Artichoke salad

Ingredients:

- **Artichokes (about 6) 1 kg**
- **Lemons for acidulated water 1**

FOR THE CITRONETTE

- **Lemon juice 30 g**
- **Salt to taste**
- **Black pepper to taste**
- **Extra virgin olive oil 60**

Start by cleaning the artichokes: prepare the acidulated water to store the artichokes without oxidizing them as you clean them. Fill a bowl with water and squeeze the juice of 1 lemon inside. Remove part of the stem of the artichokes and the more leathery leaves. With a knife cut off the tip and the outermost part of the stem to keep the inside tender. Clean the artichoke, divide it into two equal parts, thinly slice the artichokes, and place them in the bowl with acidified water as you cut them. Once the cleaning is finished, put them to drain in a colander. In the meantime, take care of the seasoning.

Squeeze 30 g of lemon juice and add it to 60 g of olive oil, salt and mix the emulsion with a whisk. Pour the artichokes into a bowl and flavor them with the citronette, mix and then serve the salad on the serving dishes!

7) Breadcumb Potatoes

Ingredients:

- **Potatoes 1 kg**
- **2 sprigs rosemary**
- **Bread crumbs 50 g**
- **Sage 3 leaves**
- **Extra virgin olive oil to taste**
- **Salt to taste**

Peel the potatoes and cut them into wedges, then place them in a bowl with water so as not to blacken them. Meanwhile, finely chop the sage, rosemary, and set aside. Now take the breadcrumbs and the chopped herbs. Now drain the potato wedges with a strainer and pour the chopped breadcrumbs and season with a drizzle of olive oil and salt.

Stir and pour into a baking tray lined with parchment paper and cover the potatoes with a spoonful of breadcrumbs. Bake the potatoes in a static oven at 180 ° for 40 minutes (if the oven is at 160 ° for 30 minutes). When cooked, your potatoes will be golden and crispy, take them out of the oven and let them cool before serving.

8) Crunchy salad

Ingredients:

- **Iceberg salad 1 large head**
- **Parmigiano Reggiano one piece or in flakes 80 g**
- **Carrots 2**
- **4 slices sandwich bread**
- **Chopped parsley 3 tbsp**
- **Anchovies fillets 8**
- **Lemon juice**
- **Salt to taste**
- **Extra virgin olive oil 2 tablespoons for frying, plus q.s. to season**

Wash the iceberg salad leaves, cut them finely, and put them in a large salad bowl. Now pass the carrots and with a potato peeler cut the carrots finely with a potato peeler; always with the potato peeler, do the same also with the Parmesan cheese.

Chop the anchovy fillets and parsley and place them in a bowl with oil, salt and mix everything with a fork and leave them for a few minutes to rest. Take the slices of sandwich bread, remove the darker edges, and cut them into 1 cm cubes on each side.

 In a pan, add two tablespoons of extra virgin olive oil, heat it and then throw it into the cubes of bread over moderate heat, turning them on all sides. Once golden, place them on absorbent kitchen paper 11. Add the carrots, Parmesan, and the oil and parsley dressing to the iceberg salad. Mix the ingredients and then add the crispy croutons 15. Ready-made salad!

9) Ginger gourd

Ingredients:

- **Pumpkin 1 kg**
- **Fresh ginger 40 g**
- **Leeks 1**
- **Vegetable broth 500 ml**
- **Extra virgin olive oil 20 g**
- **Salt to taste**

Let's start by cleaning the pumpkin, cut it in half, empty it of the seeds and internal filaments, remove the peel, and cut it into cubes. And cut it into small cubes. Wash the leek, peel it and keep the white part of the stem that you will slice in thin slices. Place a large pan on the heat, pour the leeks and season with the olive oil and fry until the leek is wilted (about 5 minutes).

At this point, pour a ladle of hot broth and add the ginger and the pumpkin cubes and salt. Pour another ladle of broth and cook over medium heat for about 25-30 minutes, adding broth little by little during cooking so as not to dry the vegetables too much. When the pumpkin is soft, turn off the heat.

The ginger pumpkin is ready to be brought to the table.

10) Roasted carrots with pistachio

Ingredients:

- **Carrots 650 g**
- **Unsalted pistachios 80 g**
- **Rosemary 3 sprigs**
- **Salt to taste**
- **Extra virgin olive oil to taste**

Wash the carrots, peel them, divide them in half and then make some sticks by cutting them for the long side. Pour the carrots into a bowl and season with rosemary, olive oil, and salt. Now roughly chop the pistachios with a knife.

Add the pistachios to the carrots and mix them to amalgamate all the ingredients. Line a baking sheet with parchment paper and pour the carrots trying to distribute them evenly in order to facilitate cooking. Bake in a preheated static oven at 220 ° for 30 minutes. Once cooked, take the roasted carrots out of the oven and let them cool before serving.

Chapter 8: Recipes for dessert

1) Cocoa pudding

Ingredients:
- **500 ml of soy milk**
- **4 tablespoons of unsweetened cocoa**
- **3-4 tablespoons of brown sugar**
- **2 tablespoons of corn starch**
- **1 pinch of natural vanilla**
- **1 pinch of ground cinnamon**
- **chopped hazelnuts to decorate**

Sift the cocoa, starch, and sugar; collect them in a saucepan together with cinnamon and vanilla. First, add 100 ml of milk, stirring well to remove all lumps, and then the rest. Over medium heat, bring to a boil without stopping stirring. Lower the heat and cook for a couple of minutes more until the mixture has thickened. Moisten four single-portion molds and pour the pudding. Let it cool down and put it in the fridge until completely cooled. Decorate with the grains and serve.

2) Baked stuffed apples

Ingredients:
- **6 apples**
- **1 orange**
- **¾ cup of shelled walnuts**
- **¾ cup of raisins**
- **¼ cup of natural apple juice**
- **1 tablespoon of miso**

Wash and with a knife, starting from the top of the apple, make room for the filling. Heat the oven to 150 °. Rinse the raisins and chop them with the walnuts. Wash the orange and finely grate the zest. Add the orange zest, miso, and a teaspoon to the raisin and nut mixture. Mix well. Stuff the apples with the dough. Arrange the apples in a baking dish. Pierce them with a fork all around so that they do not explode during cooking. Pour the apple and orange juice into the pan and bake in the oven for half an hour. Eat them warm or cold.

3) Spiced apple pie

Ingredients:
- 3 apples
- 200 g of spelled flour type 0
- 30 g of corn starch
- 50 g of raisins
- 50 g of peeled and chopped almonds
- 150-200 ml of almond or soy milk
- 120 ml of concentrated apple juice
- 50 ml of corn oil
- ½ teaspoon of cinnamon
- ½ teaspoon of vanilla
- 1 pinch of clove powder
- the grated zest of ½ lemon
- ½ sachet of baking powder
- 1 pinch of salt

Cut the apples into small pieces, soak the raisins. In a bowl, mix the flour, starch, almonds, spices, lemon peel, salt, and yeast; in another, milk, concentrated juice, oil, apples, and drained raisins. Mix all the ingredients, transfer the mixture into a pan lined with parchment paper and bake at 190 ° for about 45 minutes. Check the cooking with a toothpick before serving.

4) Carrot cake

Ingredients:
- **200 g of wholemeal flour**
- **80 g of almonds**
- **80 g of raisins**
- **200 g of carrots**
- **100 g of rice malt**
- **4 tablespoons of sunflower oil**
- **1 orange**
- **3 tablespoons of corn starch**
- **1 teaspoon of yeast**
- **½ teaspoon of natural vanilla**
- **soya milk**
- **1 pinch of salt**

Wash the orange, grate the zest and squeeze the juice. Put the first in a bowl together with the flour, finely ground almonds, starch, yeast, vanilla, and salt. Stir. Mix the oil, malt, and orange juice in a bowl. Gradually add them to the dry ingredients. Complete with grated carrots and rinsed raisins. If the dough is too firm, dilute it with a little soy milk. Line a square mold of about 20 cm on each side with baking paper. Transfer the mixture, level it, and bake at 180 degrees for about 45 minutes. Check the cooking with a toothpick, which must come out dry. Let the cake cool in the pan, turn it out of the mold, and let it cool.

5) Banana dessert

Ingredients:
- **50 g of pitted dates**
- **10 g of sultanas**
- **100 g of Pecan nuts**
- **50 g of peeled almonds**
- **50 g of Rapè coconut**
- **Himalayan salt**
- **1 tablespoon of orange juice**
- **1 tablespoon of coconut oil**
- **cinnamon powder**

For the stuffing
- **2 large bananas**
- **420 g of cashews soaked for about 6-7 hours**
- **the juice and grated zest of ½ organic lemon**
- **150 ml of agave syrup, cooled in the freezer for about 25 minutes**
- **150 g of cocoa butter**
- **1 tablespoon of coconut oil**

To garnish
- **½ bar of dark chocolate or maple syrup or chopped hazelnuts**
- **banana slices (optional)**

Wash the dates and raisins under running water, then chop them finely in a mixer; without turning off the appliance, add the salt, orange juice, coconut oil, and cinnamon. When you have obtained a compact mixture, add the Pecan nuts and the chopped almonds in thin grains separately, complete with the Rapè coconut. Mix the dough well and roll it out on the bottom of a small cake pan (or a loaf pan), which you will have lined with baking paper. Level it well on the surface using a spatula and put it to solidify in the freezer or refrigerator.

Drain the cashews and grind them for a long time in the mixer to make them doughy. Continuing to operate, first add the lemon juice and zest, agave syrup, cocoa butter, and melted coconut oil; then add the bananas and continue until you have a soft cream. Pour it on the cooled base and place it in the freezer, so that it becomes firm. You can also divide it into individual portions. Let it cool for a few minutes before serving. Decorate with a few banana slices, if you like, or with dark chocolate cut into flakes or with maple syrup and chopped hazelnuts.

6) Almond and apricot cake

Ingredients:
- **500g of chopped apricots + other ripe ones for garnish**
- **½ cup of chopped dried apricots**
- **2 tablespoons of agar-agar**
- **2 cups of almond milk**
- **2 tablespoons of almond cream**
- **the grated zest of ½ lemon**
- **1 teaspoon of vanilla**
- **4 tablespoons of corn starch**
- **½ cup of concentrated apple juice**
- **200 g of ladyfingers**
- **Apple juice**
- **salt**

Put the fresh and dried apricots in a pot together with half a cup of water, the agar-agar, and a pinch of salt. Stirring constantly, bring to a boil, and cook for 5-10 minutes. When cooked, add the concentrated juice, then blend. Use a little almond milk to dissolve the corn starch and rest on the heat with a pinch of salt, lemon peel, and vanilla. When it is about to boil, remove it from the stove, add the almond cream and starch, and then let it boil again and turn it off. Blend the apricots, add the cream and adjust the flavor by adding, if necessary, more concentrated apple juice. Cut the ladyfingers at one end and quickly dip them in the apple juice. Arrange them standing along the edge of a mold of about 22 cm and distribute the cutouts on the bottom. Cover with the apricot cream and leave to cool for a few hours. Remove the hinge from the mold and serve the cake decorated with some halved fresh apricots.

7) Strawberry tartlets

Ingredients:
For the shortcrust pastry
- **250 g of wholemeal flour**
- **50 g of coconut butter**
- **2 tablespoons of rice flour**
- **2 tablespoons of brown sugar**
- **1 teaspoon of ground cinnamon**
- **1 pinch of pink salt**

For coverage
- **4 tablespoons of unsweetened apricot jam**
- **2 tablespoons of chopped hazelnuts**
- **½ tablespoon of lemon juice**
- **1 tablespoon of cherry, plum or apricot distillate**
- **400 g of strawberries**
- **1 sprig of mint**

Melt the coconut butter in a double boiler and let it cool. Pour it into the mixer with the other ingredients and sugar. Operate; when large crumbs begin to form, add a few tablespoons of cold water at a time, continuing to knead the dough until it collects into a ball. Wrap it in a cloth and put it in the fridge for 30 minutes.

It is using a damp brush, grease 8 molds with a diameter of 10 cm with oil. Obtain from the thinly rolled dough as many discs large enough to cover the molds' walls and the bottom. They will have to adhere everywhere. Prick the bottom with a fork. Cover each tart with a piece of parchment paper and a few dried beans. Bake at 180 degrees for 15 minutes, remove the paper and the legumes, cook them for another 5 minutes. After another ten minutes, remove them, and once cold, unmold them. Heat the jam with the distillate until it is shiny. Turn off and add the lemon juice. After a few minutes, brush part of the mixture on the bases. Wash the strawberries, dry them gently and slice them not too thin. Distribute them over the dough. Cover with the remaining jam, sprinkle the surface with the grains, and let it rest in a cool place for about an hour. Just before serving, garnish the tarts with mint leaves.

8) Chocolate with avocado and orange

Ingredients:
- 200 g of pitted dates soaked for 15 minutes
- 150 g of walnut kernels
- 150 g of white almonds
- 1 tablespoon of orange juice
- 1 tablespoon of coconut oil
- ½ teaspoon of sea salt

For the stuffing
- 5 large ripe avocados, peeled
- 100 g of coconut oil
- 1 tablespoon of white almond cream
- 50 g of melted cocoa butter
- the grated zest of ½ orange
- ½ teaspoon of vanilla powder
- 170 g of cocoa powder
- 250 g of agave syrup

To garnish
- dark chocolate grains

Soak the dates for 15 minutes. Let the maple syrup cool in the freezer for about 25 minutes. Finely grind the walnuts and almonds in the bowl of a mixer. Keep them aside. In their place, put the drained dates and purée them. Then, continuing to operate the appliance, add the salt, coconut oil, orange juice, and the previously prepared grains. When you have a compact mixture, the spread is based on a pan (or a loaf pan) lined with baking paper. Level it well with a spatula and remove it in the freezer or in the refrigerator to make it firm. Gather all the ingredients required for the filling in a mixer and start. You will need to get a well blended mixture. Pour on the solidified base and pass the cake in the refrigerator or freezer so that it hardens. Decorated with one of the proposed alternatives and served.

9) Chocolate nut and almond balls

Ingredients:
- 200 g of wholemeal flour
- 150 g of walnuts
- 50 g of pine nuts
- 50 g of sunflower seeds
- 200 g of almonds
- 50 g of flax seeds
- 100 g of raisins
- 100 g of dark chocolate in small pieces
- 400 g of rice malt
- 1 lemon
- 1 orange
- 6 tablespoons of brown sugar

Soak the raisins in warm water. In the meantime, grate the peel of a lemon and an organic orange and place them in a large bowl. Add the coarsely chopped walnuts and almonds, flax seeds, sunflower seeds, and pine nuts. Stir in the flour, chocolate, and squeezed raisins and mix well with your hands. Then add the malt and continue to mix all the ingredients with energy. Lightly moisten your hands and form medium-sized balls that you will arrange quite far from each other in a baking tray lined with baking paper. Bake for about 10-12 minutes at 180 °. Let cool before serving. Excellent served accompanied by a fragrant compote of apples and spices.

10) Chocolate truffles

Ingredients:
- 100 g of dark chocolate
- 100 g of almonds
- 50 g of hazelnuts

- **100 g of dates**
- **50 g of bitter cocoa**

Soak the almonds in a glass jar for at least 3 hours, then add the dates and leave them for another hour. Meanwhile, heat the dark chocolate in a bain-marie. Drain and set aside the almond and date water. We combine the melted chocolate in the jar with the dried fruit and work it all with the hand blender. Incorporate the chopped hazelnuts and place them in the fridge for an hour. If the mixture is too hard, wet it with one or two tablespoons of soaking liquid. We sprinkle the cocoa on a saucer. We take small doses of the mixture and let them fall on the cocoa. We form balls and compact them well, trying to press them as much as possible. Let's put them in small bowls and skewer each ball with a wooden stick.

11) Tuna sauce

Ingredients:
- **100 g of tuna in oil**
- **50 g of pickled capers**
- **2 anchovies**
- **1 firm yolk**
- **the juice of 1/2 lemon**
- **1 glass of extra virgin olive oil**
- **salt**
- **pepper**

To make the tuna sauce, start chopping the tuna well drained from the oil and collect it in the mixing bowl together with the rinsed and squeezed capers, the boned anchovies, and the crumbled hard-boiled egg yolk. Soften the dough with a few tablespoons of oil and operate the appliance with short interrupted clicks. Gradually add the rest of the oil and blend for a few seconds until the desired density is obtained. Add the lemon juice filtered through a colander and mix very well. Taste and, if necessary, season with salt and pepper. Let it sit for 10 minutes. If the sauce is too thick, dilute it with a little oil. Then pour the tuna sauce in a gravy boat or a serving bowl and serve.

Chapter 9: Drinks&Shakes

1) Golden milk

Ingredients:

- **Water 130 g**
- **Turmeric powder 40 g**
- **Black pepper 1 pinch**
- **FOR A GOLDEN MILK CUP**
- **Vegetable milk (almond or soy) 150 g**
- **honey 1 tbsp**

To prepare the golden milk, you have to start with turmeric paste. Pour the water in a saucepan together with a little pepper and bring to a boil. As soon as the water boils, turn off the heat and add the turmeric powder. Stir until you have a thick and grainy paste. Finally, transfer the turmeric paste to a jar in which you can store it. Now move on to the preparation of your cup of golden milk. In a saucepan, bring the vegetable milk to a boil and then transfer it to a jar and add a teaspoon of turmeric paste, then sweeten with honey and close the jar with the cap. Ready for your golden milk!

2) Banana milkshake

Ingredients:

- **Bananas 300 g**
- **Ice 60 g**
- **Cinnamon sticks 2 g**
- **Whole milk 150 g**

To prepare the banana smoothie, we start by cutting the bananas into chunks and inserting them in the mixer. Also, add the cinnamon, not too many ice cubes, and the milk at a standing temperature.

Operate the mixer until a thick and creamy mixture is obtained. Then pour it into the glasses and decorate with a few pieces of cinnamon. The milkshake is ready.

3) Yogurt smoothie

Ingredients:

- **Yogurt 250 g**
- **Lime juice (about 1) 13 g**
- **Pulp melon 420**
- **Pulp peaches 350**

Let's start by washing the peaches (it will take about 3), peel them, and remove them from the core, then cut them into coarse pieces and set them aside. Now the melon: cut it in half, remove the seeds and peel and cut it into pieces.

Cut the lime in half and squeeze it. Collect the juice obtained in a glass and keep it aside. Now take a blender and put the and melon. Pour the yogurt and lime juice, close the blender, and activate it. Keep blending until the mixture is creamy. Your yogurt smoothie is ready!

4) Almond milk

Ingredients:

- **Peeled almonds 200 g**
- **Water 1 l**
- **Acacia honey 85 g**

To prepare almond milk, first put the almonds in a bowl with 500 g of water for at least an hour to soak. After the hour, pour both the almonds and the water into a mixer, then add the remaining 500 g of water and honey. Blend everything until a homogeneous cream is obtained, then filter the mixture obtained through a narrow mesh strainer and refrigerate for at least an hour, covered with plastic wrap. Serve your almond milk cold or at room temperature.

5) Homemade tropical fruit juice

Ingredients:

- **450 g of pineapple**
- **250g mango**
- **2 oranges**
- **1 grapefruit**
- **1.2 liters of water**
- **100g of sugar**

Start by peeling the mango and cutting it into cubes. Peel the pineapple by cutting the ends first then in half and finally in four parts. Remove the central hard part and also make the cubes pineapple. After this, extract the juice of an orange and a grapefruit.

Now transfer the citrus juice and fruit cubes to the pot with water and sugar and cook for 15 minutes. Pass 15 minutes with a hand blender and whisk until you have a puree, and you will put them in sterilized glass jars. Close the jars and put them and put them in the refrigerator until the jars cool down. They are now ready to be tasted!

6) Non-alcoholic melon cocktail

Ingredients:

- **1 untreated lemon**
- **20 grams of sugar**
- **2 slices of melon**
- **2 slices of white melon**
- **400 milliliters of carbonated mineral water**

Rinse the lemon and peel without throwing away the zest. Divide the lemon in half, squeeze it, and filter the juice obtained by passing it in a colander. Put the filtered juice and the lemon zest in a saucepan together with 20 grams of sugar. Cook everything for 2 minutes on low heat, stirring.

Filter the syrup obtained and let it cool. Peel the melon and the white melon, remove the seeds and the white filaments. Cut the pulp of the melons into small pieces. Put the melon pieces in the blender until you have obtained a homogeneous mixture. Add the previously prepared syrup to the melon smoothie. Incorporate, little by little, the carbonated mineral water to your non-alcoholic cocktail.

Blend again and put them in a container or cocktail glasses and put them in the refrigerator. Leave them to cool for a quarter of an hour. When finished, decorate the glasses as desired with straws and melon slices. Serve the non-alcoholic melon cocktail still very fresh.

7) Smoothie cheesecake

Ingredients:

- **Lean cottage cheese 250 g**
- **Fresh liquid cream 250 g**
- **Icing sugar 30 g**
- **Strawberries 280 g**
- **Yellow peaches 380 g**

To make the cheesecake smoothie, first, wash the peach and strawberries, then peel the peach and cut it into pieces, transfer it to the mixer glass and blend to get a puree. Do the same operation with the strawberries, remove the green stalk, cut them into small pieces, and place in the mixer glass to blend them until you get a puree. Now pour the ricotta into a bowl, add ¾ of the fresh liquid cream, the icing sugar and blend everything with the immersion mixer to obtain a homogeneous cream. Now add the remaining fresh liquid cream and mix to mix.

Now make your own cheesecake smoothie. Use glasses of about 70 cl capacity. The smoothie is made up of a layer of ricotta cream alternated with fruit puree. Pour the first layer of cream, move the glass slightly between your hands to evenly distribute the first layer on the bottom, cover with peach or strawberry puree, then pour a layer of ricotta cream again and finish with the strawberry or peach puree. Serve your cheesecake smoothie fresh!

8) Apple cider

Ingredients:

- **700 grams of apples**
- **50 grams of sugar**
- **100 ml of water**
- **1 orange**
- **1 lemon**
- **2 cloves**
- **1 cinnamon stick**
- **1 fresh ginger**

To prepare the apple cider, start by cutting and squeezing the orange and obtaining the juice. Do the same with the lemon. Now wash, peel, and remove the core from the apples. At this point, cut the apples until they are cubed and put in the blender until the juice is obtained, then filter it with a strainer.

Now add the sugar and the orange and lemon juice and mix so as to mix all the flavors. Now add the fresh ginger, the cloves, the cinnamon, and cook for 10 minutes. Pass the 10 minutes and filter everything, and your apple cider is ready!

9) Chai latte

Ingredients:

- **200 ml milk**
- **200 ml water**
- **2 black tea bags**
- **1 pinch of cinnamon**
- **1 pinch of cardamom**
- **2 ginger sticks**
- **1 teaspoon maple syrup**

Start by putting the water in a saucepan and bring it to a boil. Once the water boils, turn off the stove and insert the tea bags and spices. After a couple of minutes, remove the tea bags and keep them brewing for another 4 minutes.

In the meantime, take another saucepan and pour milk and a teaspoon of maple syrup. With a wooden spoon, mix well until the syrup has completely drained. You can now add the infusion in the milk and mix well to mix the flavors. Ready!

10) Fruit and yogurt cocktails

Ingredients:

- **25 gr of strawberries**
- **25 gr of raspberries**
- **125 ml of cold milk**
- **125 ml of Cold Natural Yogurt**
- **1 Teaspoon Rose Water**
- **1/2 teaspoon of light honey**

To prepare it, put the milk, strawberries, raspberries, yogurt, rose water in the blender, and blend for about 30 seconds, mixing the ingredients well. Pour into a tall drink glass, mix and add the honey. Decorate with strawberry slices or a sprig of mint, serve immediately.

Conclusion

GERD is a disorder related to the stomach and digestive system that creates irritation. The main reason behind this problem is poor nutrition, poor digestion, lack of sleep, and an incorrect lifestyle. Weight gain and other health complications can cause acid reflux. With GERD, heartburn is felt, and there is a feeling that food is coming back from the stomach.

The treatments to combat GERD in the initial phase is the correct intake of food, exercise, and following a healthy diet trying to reduce weight. If not treated well, it can cause further serious health complications such as cancer or ulcers. To get quick relief from GERD, you need to adopt some lifestyle changes such as taking small meals instead of full meals, following an exercise routine, reducing, limiting the intake of spicy and fried foods, and reducing. In the initial phase of GERD, it can be treated and prevented with healthy and organic food choices. Also, carry out an adequate medical check-up; this will help you find out how serious the problem is. Consult your family doctor and listen to his or her treatment recommendations and precautions. This is the first step you need to take to treat GERD. In this book, a series of healthy and organic recipes are mentioned that will help you finally enjoy good food and relief even in acid reflux conditions.